The Mystical Chakra Mantras

How to tune your own charkas with Mantra Yoga

The Mystical Chakra Mantras

How to tune your own charkas with Mantra Yoga

Harrison Graves MD

The Mystical Chakra Mantras

Copyright 2014 by Harrison Graves

Cover: *Stairway to OM*, from CanStockPhoto.com.

OM Channel videos by Harrison Graves

Dedication and Gratitude

I dedicate this book to Mantrakaya Sarasvati... my partner in music and mantra, and in Artha, Kama, Dharma and Moksha.

I also dedicate this book to my two amazing sons, John and Chris, who give *me* inspiration when the going gets tough. You are the bravest men I know.

I send a big "Muchas Gracias" and a hug to Janet Hosmer, for being my brilliant editor and for being such a supporter of our kirtan band, OM Nation. You are an amazingly talented woman and a guiding light in the metaphysical world.

I'm also grateful to yogini Maddy Epstein for her loving support and her feedback on the manuscript and the videos.

Thank you, Russill Paul, for transmitting the mantras to me and for being my Yoga of Sound mentor. More importantly, thank you for bringing the YOS to the West.

I also send heartfelt gratitude to my Kundalini Yoga teacher and friend, Dharmanidhi Sarasvati, founder of The Jnana Agni (Wisdom Fire) School of Yoga in Berkeley, California.

Finally, thank you, Dr. David Frawley, and Dr. Thomas Ashley-Farrand, for your wonderful books on Ayurveda and Mantra Yoga, and to Ravi Singh and Ana Brett for your DVDs on Kundalini Yoga.

Table of Contents

Preface

This book is a wonderful primer for anyone interested in chakras and mantras.

Thoughtfully written for beginner as well as advanced students, the author, Dr. Harrison Graves, explains mantras and the chakras in plain English.

It then becomes easy to understand how the mantra system works on the chakra system.

What makes this book unique, however, are its companion YouTubes on the OM Channel, where you can chant along with the author.

Dr. G. has traded in his Western specialty, Emergency Medicine, for an Eastern one: the Yoga of Sound, the yoga of music and mantra. The Yoga of Sound is an important part of Ayurveda, the holistic medicine from India. It is the fastest way to achieve the original goal of yoga… "calming the thought waves of the mind."

Mantrakaya Sarasvati
April 2014

Introduction

Namaste.

Welcome to this interactive book on the chakra mantras.

Interactive? Because of the links to the companion videos on YouTube (The OM Channel), where you can learn how to chant.

This book comes in two versions:

an e-book version, where E-readers will find individual hyperlinks to for each mantra, and… this print edition, where readers may find the mantras online, using the following webpage:

youtube.com/user/OMchannel108/videos

It is a simple book, designed with the beginner in mind, although my hope is that advanced students will enjoy it too. Here you will find easy-to-understand answers to these three questions and more:

1. What is the chakra system, and why is it so important?

2. What makes Sanskrit mantras unique?

3. What Sanskrit mantras are used to tune (activate and balance) the chakras?

As a bonus, in Chapter 4, I will introduce you to the Yoga of Sound, the much larger system of sound healing of which the chakra mantras are an important part.

Finally, I'll end the book with my prescription for you, a recommended home practice, or mantra sadhana.

As a medical doctor, I used to prescribe pills.

As a mantra yoga practitioner, I now prescribe mantras.

I go straight to the healing mantra appropriate for the condition.

According to Dr. David Frawley, "Mantras are *important medicines in themselves*, and have been lauded as such since Vedic times."

I predict that one day mantra yoga will become the new psychiatry, a path back to wellness and happiness without prescription drugs and their side effects.

I believe that chanting these mantras will help you to achieve one of the main goals of yoga: peace of mind… becoming more *sattvic*… more serene, balanced and harmonious.

Chapter 1
Mantras

"Mantras are asanas for your mind."

Dr. David Frawley

What is a mantra? The general meaning of mantra, of course, is a word or phrase repeated over and over, mentally or out loud. A *Sanskrit* mantra, however, is something special.

Sanskrit is the mystical language of ancient India. Unlike other languages, Sanskrit is based on the science of sound vibration. Word meanings are secondary. The most important thing is the effect of the sound vibration itself on the body and the mind. The best example of a Sanskrit mantra is AUM. The sound vibrations produced by chanting AUM create feelings of calmness and harmony in *all the cells* of the body.

AUM is yogic Xanax.

Man-tra comes from the Sanskrit words manas, meaning mind, and tra, meaning tool. Mantras are some of the most important tools in our yogic toolbox.

Common Misconception:

A mantra is a special phrase that must kept secret and can only be given by a guru.

Truth: The most important Yoga of Sound mantras are not secret. They can be chanted by anyone, though proper training is essential, as with hatha yoga.

5

How Sanskrit Mantras Work

In any tradition, mantras work on the basis of two powerful forces: *sound waves* and *thought waves* (intentions).

What is the secret of Sanskrit sound waves that allows us to tap into a hidden energy source?

Sanskrit was the language of India thousands of years ago, and is still the language of mantra today. There is a mystical power contained in each of the fifty letters of the Sanskrit alphabet. Each letter contains a sonic code, a healing sound vibration *unto itself*. Each of the fifty letters when repeated aloud, sends a healing energy to the chakra system of the energy body, and to the physical body as well.

It's like acupuncture with sound waves!

Sanskrit mantras have the power to energize, calm or heal. When the Sanskrit vowels and consonants are *combined* into words like AUM, they become even more powerful sound formulas that affect the entire being... body-mind and Soul.

Some mantras, like the Triambakam (Chapter 4), are for physical healing. Others, like OM Shanti, create mental peace. Still others, like the Chakra Mantras, work directly on the astral (energy) body to activate and balance the energy centers.

Mantra therapy is one of the main tools for achieving the original aim of yoga, "calming the thought waves of the mind."

Chakra Tuning: The Chakra Mantras

There are specialized mantras that tune (energize and balance) the chakras, the energy centers in the body. If your chakras are out of tune, chances are your life will be out of tune as well.

Hot Tip: The Chakra Mantras have no literal meaning.

Think of these mantras as powerful sounds, created by your own voice box, with one purpose: to energize and balance the chakras. Remember, in Sanskrit, the meaning of words is secondary. The effect of the sound vibration is much more important.

The best known Sanskrit mantra is AUM. AUM is the most important mantra and the source of all other mantras. In fact, if you want to learn just one mantra, make it AUM.

AUM is not only chanted for peacefulness and harmony, but also, on a mystical level, it is the chakra mantra for the third eye, the sixth chakra, the eye of intuition.

Here is the complete list of the seven chakras, along with their activation mantras:

Root Chakra (Moo-la-dha-ra)	Lam
Sacral Chakra (Swa-dhis-thana)	Vam
Abdominal (Mani-pura)	Ram
Heart (Ana-ha-ta)	Yam
Throat (Vi-shud-dhi)	Hum
Third Eye (Ajna)	AUM
Crown (Sa-has-ra-ra)	(Silence)

The Many Layers of AUM

AUM or OM?

AUM is often seen abbreviated as OM, especially when used as a prefix for another mantra, like OM Shanti. In this book, AUM and OM are used interchangeably. In Sanskrit, "au" has an "o" sound.

"A-U-M" reminds us that AUM is like a three-syllable word:

> Ahhhhh
> Uuuuuuuuu
> Mmmmmmmm

The three parts of A-U-M reflect the three stages of the Universe, the macrocosm:

> the beginning (Big Bang)
> the middle (the now)
> the end

Similarly, here on earth, in the physical body, the microcosm, A-U-M reflects:

> birth
> life
> death

A-U-M also relates to the three states of consciousness:

> waking
> dreaming
> deep sleep

In yoga, there is a fourth state, turiya, divine rapture, or the transcendental state. It can be found in the meditative silence that follows AUM chanting. AUM chanting won't lead to turiya overnight. That takes time. Remember, every journey starts with a first step.

AUM chanting is the best meditation, and the best *medication*, for this new millennium.

Why?

People are stressed out!

Worried. Anxious.

90% of the population cannot sit and meditate.

However, anyone can chant.

One of the main purposes of chanting mantras is to calm the mind so that seated meditation becomes possible. Before I discovered chanting, the mere thought of sitting still for meditation made me squirm. After chanting, meditation became easy.

AUM and Amen

Physicists know the Universe was born from one gigantic sound vibration. The Big Bang was a Big AUM, a sound that still reverberates 14 billion years later. AUM is the one song sung by the Universe (Uni-verse = One Song).

Over time, the sound energy became light energy, which cooled and transformed into matter, the elements, the planets.

AUM is our common heritage. It is a sound important to millions of people, even today.

The Hindu/Buddhist AUM became A(u)men in the Christian and Jewish traditions, and Amin in the Muslim tradition... meaning "of one accord."

AUM is the sound of oneness, the sound that unites us all. Chanting AUM connects humans back to their Cosmic Source in a real way.

AUM Chanting and Yoga Class

Yoga classes around the world start each class by chanting *AUM (OM)* three times.

Many end each class with *OM Shanti... Shanti... Shan-ti-hi* (Peace, Peace, Peace).

Chanting OM Shanti creates a deep feeling of peacefulness on all levels: peace of mind, peace of body, and peace of Spirit. It is soothing to the nervous system.

In each yoga class, the asanas (poses) are much more than stretching. The asanas strengthen every muscle in the body, tone the inner organs, and lead the body into a deep relaxation.

Likewise, mantras strengthen the *mind* and lead it into deep relaxation. "Mantras are asanas for your mind."

AUM and the Chakra Mantras

AUM is most often thought of as a tool to calm the mind. In this book, however, AUM is also used as the mantric key that opens the third eye (the sixth chakra). The third eye is called the eye of intuition... the eye that sees what the two physical eyes cannot. It is this inner vision that is able to see into the future, or communicate telepathically.

Note:
Third eye openings of the Hollywood variety rarely occur in real life. Most people experience a gradual increase in awareness and intuition. For example, the phone rings and you "know" who is calling, or a loved one dies far from home, and you somehow "know" it, without being told. Answers come without using Google.

Also, when the third eye opens, the sound of AUM is often heard spontaneously.

* * *

Now that we know more about mantras, let's take a closer look at the chakras, and see how the mantra system works on the chakra system.

As we go along, remember that proper Sanskrit pronunciation is critical to get the desired results, the fruit, of any mantra.

Listening to the mantras via the OM Channel links is highly recommended. E-readers will find links for home practice throughout the e-book version, so we can chant these mantras together.

Print readers: Chant along with "The Cosmic AUM" online at: youtube.com/user/OMchannel108/videos.

Chapter 2
A Journey Through the Chakras

Hot Tip: The chakras are found in the energy body (the astral body), not the physical body.

What are the Chakras?

You may have read that the chakras are the seven energy centers that lie along the spine. But what does that really mean?

It took me years to understand the chakras. The chakras seemed so foreign to me at first because they are not found in the physical body. The key was to first understand the energy (astral) body, called the acupuncture body in Chinese medicine.

The chakras (energy centers) and the meridians (channels or nadis) are key parts of this energy body in both Chinese medicine and Ayurveda, the holistic medicine from India.

The Astral Body

The energy (astral) body is our subtle body in life, and the part of our body-mind-spirit that survives death. We know the physical body will eventually decay, but what will happen to the mind, and the Spirit?

Fortunately, the mind's worries and hurries will not survive death either, any more than the physical body does. Only the Spirit, a conscious energy, survives.

This is the real you, and not your body or your personality. The real you is a Spirit, a being of light variously called the Astral Body, the Atman, the Higher Self, or the Soul Self. The natural characteristics of this Soul Self are highest awareness combined with energy… the energy of love.

You are cosmic consciousness and it's creative power, even though some days you may not feel like it.

But what is consciousness? Simply put… awareness. Cosmic consciousness is the highest awareness, the highest intelligence, the highest knowledge, the highest potential.

The Chakras and the Astral Afterlife

In my freshman year at the Medical College of Georgia in 1973, Eastern medicine had not yet penetrated the walls of most Southern medical schools. However, in 1975, consciousness pioneer Raymond Moody MD, also of MCG, wrote *Life After Life,* a book based on the near-death experiences (NDE's) of 150 patients. In his book, Dr. Moody's 150 patients told him what it is like to die.

When the physical body dies, the astral body separates. It observes what is happening from the point of view of a witness. There is no pain, and no fear of death. Most patients experience overwhelming feelings of peacefulness and well-being.

Dr. Moody's book affected me deeply. As a physician who was witnessing births and deaths with some regularity, I had more than a little curiosity about the afterlife.

Life After Life eventually became an international bestseller and has sold over 13 million copies, popularizing the subject of NDE's and astral bodies.

The Chakra System

Let's now take a closer look at the chakra system, which lies along the "spine" of the astral body.

The first chakra, the root, located at the bottom of the spine, is our point of connection with the Earth.

The seventh chakra, at the crown, is our point of connection with the Divine.

The first five chakras (root, sacral, abdominal, heart & throat) are energy transmitting and receiving stations, distributing their particular type of energy through channels called nadis in yoga, or meridians in acupuncture. Prana (life force energy, or Chi) flows from the chakras through the meridians like water through a garden hose, nurturing the entire body with a healing energy.

The sixth chakra, the third eye, is the command center, the brain of the energy (astral) body.

The charkas (literally "wheels" in Sanskrit) are like multicolored spinning pinwheels of energy.

After years of study, I realized the easiest way to understand these energy centers is to start with two chakras that are already quite familiar: the heart center and the sacral (sex) center.

The Heart Center

Perhaps the chakra most universally known is the heart center. It contains one of the the most powerful energies of all, the energy of loving kindness... the power of love. It is the energy that nourishes and protects... like a mother's love.

On the physical level, the heart chakra corresponds to the heart and lungs. The energy heart, however, is the feeling heart, the heart full of compassion. The energy heart can send out an electromagnetic wave of loving kindness so strong it can be felt across a room. When you hear the words, "I love you," *where* in the body do you feel it?

The chest, the heart center.

Sacral Chakra: The Sexual Energy Center

The Sacral Chakra is perhaps the most glamorized of energy centers... from Cosmo magazine to MTV.

Sometimes called the Sex Chakra, it is simply home to the organs of reproduction in the physical body and home of the sexual *energy* in the energy body.

In Indian philosophy, sex is not "good, bad, right or wrong." On the contrary, sexual love (Kama) is celebrated as one of the four goals of life: *Kama* (love), *Artha* (wealth), *Dharma* (compassionate service) and *Moksha* (immortality).

However, sometimes the sex chakra train goes off the track. What are the signs of a Sacral Chakra out of balance, a sex chakra out of tune?

An imbalance here can manifest as a life that is either too *promiscuous* or too *puritanical*.

Sex can attract a great deal of energy and interest, even to the point of obsession. Sexual websites were among the first to be profitable on the web. In a society where sex is wildly popular, an alien visitor might conclude the sacral chakra is the most important!

The *other* side of the sex center coin is being too *puritanical*. Suppression of the sexual energy can lead to anxieties, frustration, bitterness and depression. One definition of depression is "stuck energy" … energy that needs to move.

 When the ego mind is in charge, compulsions of all sorts can hijack the energy train. However, when the ego mind has let go, the Higher Self is in charge, and one can *choose* where to put his or her energy. That's where chakra mantras come in as they are used to direct and balance our energies. Without balance, it can be easy for the energy to become "stuck" in one chakra or another.

Balanced chakras help keep us on the right track. With a little practice, it is possible to play the chakras like a xylophone, to choose where we wish to put our energies. Then it becomes possible for the sexual energy to be used, *consciously*, for one of three purposes: procreation, recreation or higher consciousness.

According to Yogi Ravi Singh, one of the goals of yoga is to use energy wisely, like an energy-saving appliance… to "use energy consciously, not compulsively."

Brahmacharya

Some yogis make a conscious choice to practice brahmacharya, the foregoing of sex, either for short or long periods of time. Brahmacharya is more than simple abstinence, however. Its purpose is to sublimate the sexual energies to the higher chakras… to use that energy for heart's love (fourth chakra), artistic creativity (fifth chakra) or selfless service (dharma).

This sublimation (going from the mundane energies to the "sublime") often occurs naturally as the sex hormones decline. A de-emphasis of the sex chakra is often normal with aging, as the energies are naturally focused elsewhere.

* * *

Now we have touched on chakras two and four, the sex chakra and the heart chakra, let's move on to the others. They may sound surprisingly familiar, too.

To make our journey through the chakras even more intriguing, let's take a trip to a Chakra Island where we'll find interesting examples of all seven chakras and their energies.

Chakra Island

First Chakra (Root)

Pretend you just washed ashore on a remote island, much like Tom Hanks in "Castaway."

Where will you put your energy that first day?
Survival, of course.

Not sex. Not love.
Survival.

A trained survivalist will look for shelter first, then water, then food... in that order.

The first chakra, the root, located at the base of the spine, is home to this extremely powerful energy. In a life or death situation, survival energy automatically takes over and becomes paramount.

However, too much energy "stuck" in the first chakra creates an imbalance that leads to ungroundedness... to worries and anxieties, especially worries about obtaining the basic needs... food, shelter and financial security. In the extreme, this ungroundedness leads to an us-versus-them mentality, a sure sign of root chakra imbalance.

In this age of greediness and wars, it could be said that much of planet Earth's energy is stuck in the first chakra. With the evolution of consciousness, war and greed (us-versus-them) will be replaced by love and compassion (sharing and finding the win-win).

Sounds, Colors and Elements

As we journey through the chakras, remember that each chakra not only has its own unique energy, but also an associated color, element and sound (mantra) that unlocks its power.

For example, we can chant the mantra for the first chakra, *Lam* (Lahm), for "groundedness, stability and good instincts"... all qualities that help ensure our survival, and the survival of the planet.

The color of the Root Chakra is dark red, like the Georgia clay. It is associated with earth element, the perfect metaphor for groundedness.

<u>Second Chakra (Sacral)</u>

Back on the island, where does the energy go after survival needs are met? There are several possibilities.

Pretend that, as a survivor, you are well supplied with water, coconuts, and food from the sea. All immediate needs are met. About a month later, another castaway washes ashore... a castaway with all the qualities that you adore.

You both hit it off. You feel natural with each other.

There is an immediate feeling of closeness, made even deeper by the shared ordeal.

Energy is now likely to ascend either to the second chakra, the sacral (sex) chakra, and/or the fourth chakra, the heart center, home of unconditional love. You are now sharing a sacral chakra and/or a heart chakra connection.

The mantra that activates (strengthens and balances) the sex chakra is *Vam* (Vahm).

The color here is orange, like the rising sun.

The Sacral Chakra is associated with water element, a metaphor that goes beyond sexuality to fluidity and connectivity.

Third Chakra (Solar Plexus)

You both have survived and thrived on the island.

What's next? Will you be rescued and make it back to civilization?

Should you intend to leave the island, you will need to rely on the next energy, the power of will, the fire in the belly, found in our next chakra, at the solar plexus. It is the location of our core strength, our power to achieve. It makes the impossible possible.

How do we strengthen willpower?

How do we make our third chakra strong?

Hot Tip: Willpower comes from building core strength with asana, breath practices and mantra.

The asanas (hatha yoga poses) add strength and flexibility to the body. A stronger body makes for a stronger mind.

Secondly, breath practices, like "breath of fire" can stoke up the third chakra fire. (See DVD *Kundalini Yoga* by Ravi Singh and Ana Brett for excellent instructions on the breath of fire.)

The third way to boost willpower is by chanting the chakra mantra Ram (Rahm).

The color of the solar chakra is bright yellow, like the midday sun. It is associated with fire element, e.g. the fire of purification, and the fire of transformation.

Purification here means to make more *sattvic,* or balanced. Sattva is a state of mind that is calm, steady and peaceful.

Fourth Chakra (Heart) - The Power of Love

The fourth chakra, the heart center, is the most important chakra for human beings. Ram Dass, author of *Be Here Now*, loved to say that true enlightenment is found through the heart and not the head.

It seems universally known that the heart center is all about love and compassion. Heart love is what every human craves. It is an unconditional loving kindness that is there for the long haul.

* * *

Back on the Island…
Forever bound together by their island ordeal, our castaways may become soul mates, dreaming of a lifetime together, hearts wide open.

The mantric key to the heart center is *Yam* (Yahm).
The color here is emerald green.
The associated element is air.

Like the air, love moves freely and fills up its container.

Chant *Yam* today and open the heart to love.

Fifth Chakra (Throat) - Creativity and Communication

"The most beautiful experience we can have is the mysterious. It is the source of all true art and science."
Albert Einstein

Upon first glance, the fifth chakra may not seem as familiar as the first four. It *is* more subtle. The throat chakra is the home of our creative energies, the home of self-expression, artistic endeavor, and even scientific discovery.

In the physical body, the throat chakra corresponds to the larynx, the voice box, the organ of communication.

The voice, the world's oldest musical instrument, is always with us, ready for communication, singing, music or mantra.

One of the best examples of fifth chakra expression is the poet-saint, Rumi, whose every word was pure poetry.

Three Rumi examples:

"Do not feel lonely. The entire Universe is within you."

"We've come to the place where everything is music."

"Break my heart so that my love may flow more freely!"

* * *

Who is your favorite creative genius?
Leonardo Da Vinci? Mozart? Cab Calloway?
Georgia O'Keefe? Frida Kahlo? Albert Einstein?

These are artists singing, writing, creating and inventing from a soul level. All represent throat chakras on fire with poetry, music and/or knowledge. Instead of a trickle charge, there is now access to the full power plant.

Mantras that stimulate the fifth chakra are one of the most potent ways to unleash your creative power.

The mantric key that unlocks the throat chakra is *Hum*.

The color here is sky blue.

The element is space… limitless and formless space.

Chant *Hum* today and discover your artistic self.

Tap into the art of creating, and even the art of healing.

* * *

Back on the Island, our castaways are now brimming with willpower from Ram chanting, hatha yoga and breath of fire. Feeling its time to leave the island, they may choose to put some fifth chakra energy toward a rescue.

Tapping into a newfound creativity, they may invent a seaworthy raft, like Tom Hanks did, or discover a way to make fire and smoke. They could use their voices to pray or to chant obstacle-busting mantras, both throat chakra practices that could lead to a rescue. After rescue, they may want to continue their soul growth by putting their energies into artistic pursuits, perhaps writing a book about the adventure of a lifetime.

Sixth Chakra - The Third Eye

The sixth chakra is the command center, the brain of the energy body. It is the seat of higher wisdom and intuition and the home of the psychic energy. Located between the eyebrows, it is often called the "eye of intuition."

When the third eye is open, telepathic communication becomes possible. One may become able to "see" the future, and even to connect with the "cosmic internet," the source of all knowledge.

The mantric key to the third eye is AUM.

The color of this sixth chakra is indigo.

* * *

Back on Chakra Island

Back on the island, our castaways are now able to communicate telepathically. Feelings are expressed and understood without words.

They may choose to create a rescue by sending out a telepathic SOS. Or, they could choose to go within and meditate. They could even come to the point called vairagya, equanimity in all things... being ok with rescue or non-rescue.

Meditation on the third eye, especially while chanting AUM, naturally leads to a connection with the cosmos, with the Divine.

In time, meditation will naturally and spontaneously lead to the final destination: the crown chakra and beyond.

Seventh Chakra - The Crown

Finally we come to the top of the head, the crown... the culmination of our chakra journey. It is not so much another energy center as it is our point of connection with the Divine.

Think of yourself as a AA battery. The first chakra, the flat bottom of the battery, is the point of connection with the Earth. The crown chakra, the knob at the top of the battery, is the point of connection with the Divine... the higher Self.

Another name here is Sahasrara Chakra, the thousand-petalled lotus.

The color here is the pure Light that contains all colors.

The sound here is the silence beyond sound.

When all the chakras are balanced, the kundalini energy can flow all the way up the spine to the top, to Sahasrara Chakra, leading to a feeling of connection with the Universe and with all other beings.

The crown chakra becomes especially important at the time of death. When the body dies, the consciousness exits through the crown chakra at the top of the head. The departing consciousness experiences the sensation as a journey traveling through a silver tunnel (sushumna nadi) toward a brilliant light, the Light of cosmic con-sciousness.

It is a final journey through the chakras.

Feelings of oneness, joy and deep inner peace are experienced. One feels connected with Divine Love, the Universe and all other beings. One realizes there was no need to fear the death of the physical body.

In *Autobiography of a Yogi*, Swami Yogananda goes into great detail about the astral body and astral heaven:

The physical body is replaced by a body made of light.
Astral travel is accomplished instantaneously by thoughts.
All communication is telepathic.
There is no sickness or suffering.

According to Sri Yogananda, nearly all individuals enter the Astral plane after death. There they may choose to stay in astral heaven or return to an earthly incarnation to continue the Soul's journey.

Author's note:
Steve Job's last wish was that *Autobiography of a Yogi* be handed out to all those in attendance at his funeral.

Steve's last words were, "Wow... WOW!"

Could it be that he was catching his first glimpse of astral heaven?

Summary

Each of the first six chakras has its own energy and its own mystical sound, a vibrational key that unlocks its power.

Here is the full table of the chakras, their energies and their mantras:

Chakra	Type of Energy	Mantra
Root Chakra	Survival energy	Lam
Sacral Chakra	Sexual energy	Vam
Solar	Energy of Will	Ram
Heart	Love energy	Yam
Throat	Creative energy	Hum
Third Eye	Intuitive energy	AUM
Crown	Energy of the Divine	(Silence)

Chapter 3
The Chakra Mantras

How to tune your own chakras… with the Yoga of Sound

Now that we better understand the chakras and their energies, let's focus on the chakra mantras in more detail.

The chakra mantras have three things in common:

Each activates and balances its corresponding chakra.
Each has one syllable.
Each ends with "m."

They are also called bija (seed) mantras. Just like the seed of an orange tree contains the stored energy needed to create the tree, so it is with the bija mantras. Each seed *sound* contains all the vibrational energy needed to tune (activate and balance) its corresponding chakra.

The bijas vibrationally energize their chakras like water and light energize a plant. Think of each bija as a packet of vibrational energy, a sound formula, created by your own voice. Think of them as sound vibrations that activate chakras.

Hot Tip:
The bija mantras are the simplest mantras (one-syllable) and at the same time, among the most powerful.

Let's start our sound journey with the first chakra, at the base, the root, of the spine.

Root Chakra Mantra: Lam

We learned in Chapter 2 that *Lam* (*Lahm*) is the mantra for groundedness. As we chant this mantra together, think:

I am grounded.
I am stable.
I trust my instincts.

Print Edition Readers:
Chant the mantra 9 times, slowly (over about 10 seconds):

Inhale.
Lam Lam Lam Lam
Lam Lam Lam Lam
Lammmmm

Repeat x 6

* * *

Chant "Lam" today and feel as grounded as the red Earth itself. Feel confident and say goodbye to worry.

Note: for home practice, this mantra can be found on the following webpage:

youtube.com/user/OMchannel108/videos, under "Chakra Mantra Lam."

Sex Chakra Mantra: Vam

Balancing the sex chakra in modern society can be challenging, especially for men.

What's the mantric way to tune the sacral chakra, to balance the sexual energy? Chanting *Vam* (Vahm).

When this chakra is finely tuned, the sexual energy can be used consciously, with awareness. New possibilities arise.

Print Edition Readers:
Chant slowly (over about 10 seconds):

Inhale.
Vam Vam Vam Vam
Vam Vam Vam Vam
Vammmmm

Repeat x 6

Chant Vam and become master of your universe.

Note: the mantra can also be found on the following webpage: **youtube.com/user/OMchannel108/videos**, under "Chakra Mantra Vam."

Solar Plexus Chakra Mantra: Ram

In Chapter 2, we learned the third chakra, the solar plexus is all about willpower. With enough willpower, all things become possible.

The mantric way to stoke up the fire of will is to chant *Ram* (rhymes with mom).

You can take control of your destiny right now with this powerful mantra.

Print Edition Readers:
Chant slowly (over about 10 seconds):

Inhale.
Ram Ram Ram Ram
Ram Ram Ram Ram
Rammmmm

Repeat x 6

Note: the mantra can be found on the following webpage:
youtube.com/user/OMchannel108/videos, under
"Chakra Mantra Ram."

Mahatma Gandhi chanted Ram with every breath, and
created enough iccha shakti, enough willpower, to defeat
the British Empire… not with weapons… with mantra.

Note: In India, *Ram* is a dual purpose mantra. Besides
being the bija mantra for the solar plexus, it is also used
as a devotional mantra to the avatar Rama.

Heart Chakra Mantra: Yam

The heart chakra is the home of loving kindness, like the
love of a mother or a father for a child.

Some hearts are open to giving and receiving love, others
are not. My heart was closed up like a rock at one time.
All those years as an ER doctor it was often too painful
for me to feel my feelings. What opened it back up? It
was a combination of three things: unconditional love
from my wife and sons, daily yoga, and mantric chanting.

Open your heart right now by chanting *Yam* (Yahm), as in
yummy.

Print Edition Readers:
Chant slowly (over about 10 seconds):

Inhale.
Yam Yam Yam Yam
Yam Yam Yam Yam
Yammmmm

Repeat x 6

Note: the mantra can also be found on the following webpage: **youtube.com/user/OMchannel108/videos**, under "Chakra Mantra Yam."

Chant Yam today as you visualize yourself connected, heart to heart, with all other beings.

Throat Chakra Mantra: Hum

As we move up the chakra ladder, everything becomes more subtle. So it is with the energy of the throat center. Here we find the energy of creativity and self-expression… the arts, music and mantra.

This fifth chakra is a wonderful place to put one's energy.

How well developed is your throat chakra?

Do you love to sing? To dance? To paint?

To play drums?

Have you found your artistic talent, your way of expressing yourself? Are you a writer, a poet, an inventor?

These are all throat chakra energies.

The chakra mantra for the throat center is "Hum" as in "humming." Chanting *Hum* creates space, energy and movement for new possibilities.

Start unlocking your creative genius today by chanting Hum.

Print Edition Readers:
Chant *Hum* (rhymes with thumb) slowly, over about 10 seconds.

Inhale.
Hum Hum Hum Hum
Hum Hum Hum Hum
Hummmmm

Repeat x 6

Note: the mantra can be found on the following webpage: **youtube.com/user/OMchannel108/videos**, under "Chakra Mantra Hum."

Third Eye Mantra: AUM

The most direct yogic method for opening the third eye is to chant AUM.

We know that AUM chanting can calm the thought waves of the mind... .the worries and the hurries. When the mind is calmed, the eye of intuition can open *spontaneously*.

One doesn't have to "do" anything... but chant.

One can't "make" it happen... one can, however, *let* it happen.

Chant AUM with me now… and feel more calm, harmonious and connected.

Print Edition Readers:
Chant slowly (over about 10 seconds):

Inhale.
AUM AUM AUM AUM
AUM AUM AUM AUM
Aummmmm

Repeat x 6

Note: the mantra can be found on the following webpage: **youtube.com/user/OMchannel108/videos**, under "Chakra Mantra AUM."

Crown Chakra: The Sound of Silence

What about the crown chakra, the culmination of our chakra journey? Does it have a bija mantra, a seed sound?

No.

The sound of the crown is silence.

It is a space beyond sound. It is the abode of Sat-Chit-Ananda… .truth, consciousness and bliss.

The true chakra journey consists of connecting with that highest bliss and bringing it back down to the heart.

Note: In some traditions, AUM is the chakra mantra for the crown, and Ksham the mantra for the third eye.

Putting It All Together: A Journey Through the Chakras

Now that you have been introduced to the chakra mantras and chanted them one at a time, let's put them all together in sequence as we chant our way through the chakras from the root to the crown.

Chant each mantra as you visualize a healing energy permeating each chakra:

Lam x 9
Vam x 9
Ram x 9 … etc.

This mantric meditation can be found on the following webpage: **youtube.com/user/OMchannel108/videos,** under "Chakra Mantra Meditation"
(6 minutes, 38 seconds).

Summary

We have learned how Sanskrit mantras are different from other mantras, and how the mantra system works on the chakra system.

We are now able to energize and balance our chakras with the bija mantras, each a powerful and mystical sound vibration that works directly on its corresponding chakra.

Chakra	Type of Energy	Bija Mantra
Root	Survival energy	Lam
Sacral	Sexual energy	Vam
Solar	Energy of Will	Ram
Heart	Love energy	Yam
Throat	Creative energy	Hum
Third Eye	Intuitive energy	AUM
Crown	Energy of the Divine	(Silence)

Why is it so important to keep our chakras finely tuned?

Here are seven reasons, one for each chakra:

1. Groundedness… to feel safe and secure

2. Sexual Balance… to choose where to put one's energy

3. Willpower… to determine one's own fate

4. Loving kindness… to discover the most important thing

5. Creativity… to express your true Self

6. Intuition… to tap into a higher wisdom

7. Enlightenment… to find the divinity within

Home Practice

Here is my chakra tuning **Rx** for you:

Chant the chakra mantras once a day, using the youtube "Chakra Mantra Meditation" as a guide:

youtube.com/user/OMchannel108/videos, "Chakra Mantra Meditation" (6 minutes, 38 seconds).

Daily mantric chanting doesn't just balance your chakras, it balances your life. It put's your higher Self in charge... your elder, your higher consciousness.

"Mantra is the safest, easiest and most available tool to tap into that massive reservoir of chakra energy and start the journey toward reaching your highest potential."

Dr. David Frawley

I mentioned before that the chakra mantras fit into a much larger system of sound healing called The Yoga of Sound (YOS). In the next chapter we will learn about all three components of the YOS tradition and find some fascinating examples of each.

Chapter 4
The Yoga of Sound

"Mantras bring bliss like no other spiritual practice."

Chris Reed CEO, yogi and humanitarian

The chakra mantras in this book are an important part of the Yoga of Sound tradition… a system of holistic healing from India. The YOS combines music with mantra.

Far more than OM chanting, the Yoga of Sound has three main parts:

1. Vedic mantras
2. Tantric mantras
3. Bhakti mantras

Let's take a brief look at all three.

Note: The Yoga of Sound is as universal as hatha yoga, and does not belong to any one spiritual path.

1. Vedic Mantras: Power and Protection

The Vedic mantras are for power, protection and overcoming obstacles. Veda means "knowledge," ancient knowledge. Here we find the spontaneously revealed knowledge from the sages and seers of India, including the Upanishads, among the most revered of the ancient texts.

According to Swami Muktananda, Vedic chanting "removes all obstacles, calamities and afflictions, takes away the fear of death and bestows prosperity, joy and the bliss of liberation."

That's quite a list.

I start each day with the great Upanishadic chant to overcome problems, *OM Gam Ga-na-pa-ta-ye Nam-a-ha.*

It is a chant to Ganapaty (Ganesha), who in India is the patron saint of solving problems and starting new ventures. It is a Sanskrit sound formula that works in mysterious ways.

Think: "I call upon the Energy of the Cosmos to help me solve this problem."

I have used this mantra many times, for obstacles great and small, everything from finding a parking space to solving a health issue to landing a job. It has never let me down.

Problems come up each day and need to be overcome. This is the mantra to make your day s-m-o-o-t-h in every way, from that interview with the boss to that problem with a relationship.

Note: to chant along, please go to the following webpage: **youtube.com/user/OMchannel108/videos**, under "Ganesha Mantra."

Another Vedic mantra I chant every day is the Triambakam, or "Great Victory Over Death" (Maha-mrit-yun-jaya) mantra:

OM	Tri-am-ba-kam	Ya-ja-ma-he
Su-ghan-dhim	Pushti-var-dha-nam	
Ur-va	Ruk-ha-mi-va	Bhan-da-naan
Myrit-yor	Mok-shi-ya	Mam-ri-tat

Acting as a protective shield, this mantra can set up a sonic force field that keeps illness and misfortune away.

A Swami friend of mine, Nandi, told me how this mantra saved his life. He was rappelling down a cliff in South India after exploring some yogi caves there. Midway down the cliff a huge swarm of angry bees descended upon him and his climbing partner. The partner was attacked, sustaining hundreds of bee stings. Almost stung to death, he eventually recovered in the hospital.

On the other hand, Nandi was untouched. By coincidence, he had been doing a mantra sadhana (extensive mantra practice) for almost 40 days, exclusively chanting the Triambakam mantra.

His body was projecting a sonic force field. His cells were putting out a loud, vibrating "Do Not Disturb" sign!

"A Sanskrit mantra is a word which 'protects *just by the virtue of being repeated.'"*

Pandit Tigunait

Note: to chant along, please go to the following webpage:

youtube.com/user/OMchannel108/videos, "Triambakam Mantra."

More examples of Vedic chanting can be found on Russill Paul's album, *Shabda* ("The Word").

41

2. Tantric Mantras

Tantric mantras are mantras for creating and/or moving energy, and are the second part of the Yoga of Sound.

Two examples of the Tantric mantras are OM Shak-ti (to create energy), and the Chakra Mantras in this book (to distribute the energy).

OM Shak-ti and OM Shan-ti

In Chapter 1 we learned that *OM Shan-ti* is chanted for peacefulness. *Om Shak-ti,* on the other hand, has quite a different effect. It is an energizing mantra. Chanting *OM Shak-ti* creates new energy available for distribution throughout the chakra system.

In Sanskrit "Shak-ti" means energy, and it also means "goddess." In India the Goddess, the Divine Feminine, represents the cosmic energy, while the Divine Masculine represents cosmic consciousness.

3. Bhakti Mantras
(How to sing your way to Enlightenment)

The third type of mantra is the devotional, or Bhakti, mantra.

Devotional mantras from every tradition have one purpose: to open the heart to love. These are songs that cultivate deep feelings of love and devotion in the heart.

Singing devotional songs in any tradition can lead to truly mystical experiences. When we sing with deep feeling in the heart, the love and devotion we sing about enters the soul.

Bhakti Yogis literally sing their way to enlightenment.

They *become* the vibration of the sound that they repeat.

Use whatever divine names resonate in *your* heart.

If you are a Christian, sing to Jesus.
If you are Hindu, sing to Shiva or Krishna.
If you are Buddhist, sing *Om Mani Padme Hum*.
And so on.

If you are not sure what to believe in, sing *The Long Time Sun*, by Snatam Kauer (also on YouTube… over 1 million hits and counting). The URL is:

youtube.com/watch?v=T1D3ejwQiVg.

This song is nothing less than a Celtic chant for enlightenment, combined with the Sanskrit *Sat Nam*.

May the Long Time Sun Shine Upon You
All Love Surround You
And the Pure Light within You
Guide your way on.
Sat Nam.

The Long Time Sun is the divine light within each being.

Sat Nam means the "Truth Within". Sing it often enough, and the truth within reveals itself.

Bhakti, the yoga of love and devotion, has become wildly popular in the West, thanks to kirtan (devotional singing) superstars Krishna Das, Deva Premal, Donna De Lory, Larisa Stow, Jai Uttal, OM Nation and many others.

One of my favorite Bhakti yogis is Donna De Lory, kirtan queen and former backup singer for Madonna.

Feel the devotion in her voice as she sings, "Jai Ma," or "Praise to the Cosmic Mother (Durga)" , available on itunes:

Hey Ma Durga, I want to love through your love,
Hey Ma Durga, I want to feel what you feel.
Hey Ma Durga, I want to see beyond this illusion... to what is real.

Donna De Lory

* * *

An example of Bhakti music, Western style, is the Hallelujah Chorus by George Frederick Handel.
Hallelu- means "Praise."
Jah means the "Divine."

To experience this devotional song in a most unusual way, please go to YouTube for "Christmas Food Court Flash Mob", 43 million views and counting.

The URL is: **youtube.com/watch?v=SXh7JR9oKVE**.

* * *

Enlightenment

According to Dr. David Frawley, there are two general paths to enlightenment: Jnana Yoga, the yoga of knowledge and self-inquiry, and Bhakti Yoga, the yoga of love and devotion.

Bhakti yoga is by far the easiest path, and the best path for this age. There is one requirement for all Bhaktas, however. A Bhakta needs something or someone to believe in.

Some folks see the Divine as Jesus, others as a Cosmic father or mother. Some relate to the divine through a guru, a teacher or a friend. Still another option is to realize that you yourself are a Divine spark of creation, where you can worship the divinity within yourself.

* * *

Of the three branches of the Yoga of Sound, Tantric Chanting and Vedic Chanting remain virtually unknown in the West. For further information, please see *The Yoga of Sound* (both the book and a boxed set of 3 CDs) by my teacher, Russill Paul.

Note: The Sanskrit name for the YOS is Nada Yoga. Nada means "sound." For many, Nada Yoga is a spiritual path that includes not only chanting, but also classical Indian music, e.g. music by Ravi Shankar or Russill Paul.

Here we find the ragas, the intricate themes and variations of the musical scale that mirror the emotions and the chakras. It is not a coincidence that there are 7 chakras and 7 notes in the musical scale. Each note corresponds to a chakra vibration.

* * *

Mantra Q & A with Dr. G

In addition to the Chakra Mantras, what other mantras do you personally chant?

For smooth sailing every day, I do a series of chants I call the Fab Five. I chant each mantra for about two minutes and create a vibratory pattern that will overcome obstacles and set the tone for the entire day.

The Fab Five Playlist

1. *Aum*
2. *The Ganesha Mantra*
3. *Triambakam Mantra*
4. *Gayatri Mantra*
5. *Lokah Samastha*

[Note to Print Readers: See the youtube playlist at the end of the book to help you access the Fab Five online.]

With this series of chants I can connect with the Universe with AUM, blast away problems with the Ganesha mantra, put on a protective suit of armor with the Triambakam, take a few steps closer to enlightenment with the Gayatri, and say a prayer for all beings with Lokah Samastha.

This set of five Vedic Mantras is ideally chanted twice daily, once each morning and once each evening, for power, protection and for accomplishing life's four goals: Kama (Love), Artha (Prosperity), Dharma (Compassionate Service) and Moksha (Enlightenment).

Bhakti Mantras can be sung anytime to cultivate feelings of love, gratitude and devotion.

The Tantric Mantras are chanted anytime a mantra practitioner wishes to create, move or balance energy.

Do I have to sing, or can I have the mantras playing in the background to obtain benefit?

The best place to start is by listening. Then sing.

Both will be of benefit.

It is best to first chant the mantra out loud, then whispered, then silently to yourself. You will know you have "seated" the mantra when you can "hear" the mantra repeating itself like a favorite song.

Do I need to learn the Sanskrit translations?

No.

Since these mantras work on the basis of sound vibration,

the translations are not the most important thing.

Of course, knowledge of the translation will make the mantras more meaningful.

Is it best to think about the chakra matching the mantra?

Yes, when chanting the chakra mantras, it is best to visualize each chakra and its position along the spine, as you chant its healing mantra.

Make it a mantra meditation.

Closing Thoughts

In October of 2013, I attended "MantraFest On Tour" at the Olympic Theater in Montreal. The headliners were

Deva Premal, Miten, Manose, Hans Christian, Manesh de Moor and the Guru Ganesha Band.

Imagine 2000 people chanting OM together. The entire theater seemed to vibrate with feelings of peacefulness and harmony. It was a life-changing experience for me, and a sign of things to come.

Mantra meditations, music and prayers from around the world are a powerful force, bringing people together and creating more love on Earth.

Afterword
Hindu-Christian Ashram

How the Hindus and the Baptists Became One

"Religion is for those who fear Hell.
Spirituality is for those who've been there."

Miten

As mentioned in Chapter 4, The Yoga of Sound is as universal as hatha yoga. It does not belong to any one religion, though it may be a spiritual path for many.

Here is an example from my personal experience… a fascinating story of eclectic pilgrims in a South India ashram.

In 2002, my wife and I traveled to Chennai, India, on a pilgrimage hosted by Master Sound Yogi Russill Paul (Anirud Jaidev), and his wonderful wife Asha. We were among those who had chosen yoga as a spiritual path.

Our diverse group consisted of about a dozen nonconformist pilgrims, including New Agers from California, Southern Baptists from Texas, and Catholics from New England.

We stayed in the simple dorms of the universally respected ashram and spiritual center, Shantivanam ("Forest of Peace"), in Tamil Nadu, South India.

We all chanted together and shared the yummy vegetarian meals, including the rice pudding specially prepared in a fire pit for Pongal, the harvest festival celebrated each January in South India.

Shantivanam is known as a Hindu-Christian ashram... a label that would ignite fireworks in the West, but would not raise an eyebrow in India.

Hymns are sung to Jesus in the morning and to Shiva/Parvati in the evening:

"OM Namah Je-su" ...   in the morning.
"OM Namah Shi-va-ya" ...   in the evening.

It's the ultimate lesson in Oneness. In fact, the monks at Shantivanam love all the avatars, all the masters who came to Earth to help mankind. Krishna is revered as the avatar who came to Earth 3000 years before Jesus. Gautama Buddha is considered to be the avatar who came 500 years before Jesus. And Jesus is the avatar who came 500 years after the Buddha. Each time, the world was in a heap of trouble, and needed someone to show the way.

One Earth.
Many Avatars.

Whenever righteousness wanes and unrighteousness increases I send myself forth.
For the protection of the good and for the destruction of evil, and for the establishment of righteousness, I come into being age after age.
                                        Bhagavad Gita: 4.7–8

Even now, there are higher awareness beings among us. Many are chanting unceasingly, silently or out loud, to elevate the consciousness of the planet.

Happiness as a planet cannot occur until the awareness is elevated. It cannot occur until those who have wealth and health develop more awareness for those who have little.

Orphanage Ashram

During our trip to India, we visited a Spiritual Center for Yoginis, the Sri Lalita Mahila Samajam. It is an orphanage-ashram, in South India, run entirely by women monks, or "virgin yoginis." The yoginis feed and clothe 150 destitute girls, many of whom have lost one or both parents. They also run a school for 400 young women.

The yoginis chant tirelessly as they perform pujas (chanting ceremonies) to elevate the consciousness of the planet.

If you have wealth, please send a portion of it to them.

They are worthy of your generosity.

If you would like to contribute, here is a link for you to do so via Peggy Cappy, host of the PBS series *Yoga for the Rest of Us* : peggycappy.net/india1.html.

Print readers:
Peggy Cappy
P.O. Box 745
Peterborough, NH 03458

Peggy also accompanied Russill Paul on a pilgrimage to India, in 2009, and has been a prime supporter of the orphanage-ashram ever since.

Father Bede and Russill Paul

Russill Paul's Guru at Shantivanam had been Father Bede Griffiths (1906-1993), a Benedictine monk and mystic from England.

Father Bede's constant theme was universality.

His progressive views, however, created problems for him with a conservative Catholic church. He emphasized love over sin and recognized that the Divine is feminine as well as masculine. He also recommended that clergy be able to marry and that women be allowed to enter the priesthood. He embraced all religions as one.

It was radical stuff, far ahead of its time.

Under Father Bede's guidance, Russill experienced a full kundalini awakening while at Shantivanam. All chakras fully powered, he became the musical and mantra genius largely responsible for bringing the Yoga of Sound to the West.

Russill has devoted his entire life to selflessly teaching mantra yoga, and creating beautiful music. For more information, see russillpaul.com.

* * *

During our visit to India, we chanted mantras like *Lokah Samastha* (May All Beings Be Happy and Free), in some of the sacred temples of South India.

One night, my wife and I walked with Russill to a nearby funeral pyre on the sacred Cauvery River, where we chanted liberation mantras (Gayatri and Mahamrityunjaya) into the cremation fire as it consumed the dead body.

Actively participating in the transition of a freshly departed soul was an experience powerful beyond words.

* * *

Trips to India seem to always be life changing… sometimes in unexpected ways. After my trip to India, I became less and less enchanted with the world of Western medicine. At the same time, I grew increasingly interested in the benefits of alternative medicine, especially Mantra Yoga, Ayurveda and Reiki. I felt that many ailments, especially those that are stress related, could be better treated with an Eastern approach.

Ultimately I chose an encore career teaching the Yoga of Sound, as mantric chanting is one of the most important tools in Ayurveda for "calming the thought waves of the mind."

About the Author

After a 30 year career as a board-certified ER physician, including associate faculty at UNC-CH, Dr. Graves gave up his Western medical practice in order to teach mantra yoga.

His sound yoga mentor had been Russill Paul (Anirud Jaidev) of Chennai, who accepted him as a student for a one-year Yoga of Sound internship back in 2002.

After 9 years of mantra sadhana and a trip to India, he began to teach mantra yoga in area yoga studios, and, along with Mantrakaya Sarasvati, formed the kirtan band, OM Nation.

In 2014 he created the OM Channel as a YouTube companion to his books and as a global vehicle for teaching the Yoga of Sound.

His next book will be *Mystical Mantras for Anxiety and Depression.*

Note:
Dr. Graves is available to teach Yoga of Sound workshops.

He can be reached at harrisongravesmd@gmail.com.

Glossary

Ajna	The sixth (brow) chakra, or "third eye"
Anahata	The heart chakra
Artha	Wealth (one of the four goals of life)
Astral body	Energy body, or acupuncture body
AUM	Mantra for oneness and harmony, also the bija mantra for the sixth chakra.
Ayurveda	The system of holistic medicine from India
Bhakti Yoga	The yoga of love and devotion, often synonymous with devotional singing, or kirtan
Bija mantras	single syllable seed sounds, like the chakra mantras, that contain all the energy of the mantra in one word
Brahmacharya	Sublimation of the sexual energy
Chakras	The energy centers that lie along the spine; literally, "wheels"
Dharma	Compassionate service (one of life's four goals)
Durga	Fierce, yet loving form of the goddess in Indian mythology
Ganapaty	another name for Ganesha, friend of the ganas, the outcasts from society
Ganesha	In Indian mythology, the elephant-headed patron saint of problem solving
Gayatri	The mother of all mantras for enlightenment; Gayatri also means "goddess"
Hum	Bija mantra for the throat center (Vishuddhi)

Jai	"praise" (example: Jai Ma means "praise to the mother")
Kama	Love (one of the four goals of life; example: Kama Sutra, "Verses of Love")
Karma	The law of cause and effect
Lam	Bija mantra for the root chakra, Mooladhara
Ma	Ma (the Cosmic Mother)
Mantra	a word or phrase said repeatedly
Manipura	Solar plexus chakra
Moksha	Immortality, enlightenment (one of the four goals of life)
Mooladhara	First chakra (root) at the base of the spine
Nada Yoga	Sanskrit name for the Yoga of Sound
Namaste	"The divine light in me honors the divine light in you."
OM	a mantra for oneness and harmony (see AUM)
Puja	a ceremony, often with chanting and a fire
Ram	Bija mantra for the solar plexus (third chakra)
Sadhana	Daily spiritual practice
Sahasrara	The crown chakra, the point of connection with the divine
Sanskrit	The mystical language of ancient India, the language of mantra
Sattvic	balanced and harmonious
Shakti	Shakti means "energy"; Shakti also means goddess
Shanti	An important mantra for peacefulness

Swadhisthana	The Sacral Chakra (sex chakra)
Tantric mantras	Mantras for creating and moving energy
Triambakam	Vedic mantra for power and protection
Vairagya	equanimity in all things; being ok with what is
Vam	Bija mantra for the Sacral Chakra
Vedas	The oldest verses of knowledge from India, including the Upanishads.
Vishuddhi	The throat chakra
Yam	Bija mantra for the heart chakra

Bibliography

1. Ashley-Farrand, Thomas. *Healing Mantras,* New York: Ballantine Wellspring books, 1999.
------------------.*Shakti Mantras* New York: Ballantine Wellspring books, 2003.
------------------. *Chakra Mantras* San Francisco: Red Wheel/Weiser LLC, 2006.

2. Dass, Ram, *Be Here Now*, San Cristobel, New Mexico:
Lama Foundation, 1971.

3. Frawley, Dr. David, *Mantra Yoga and Primal Sound: Secrets of the Bija Mantras* Twin Lakes, Wisconsin: Lotus Press, 2010.

4. "Life After Life." In Wikipedia. http://en.wikipedia.org/wiki/Life_After_Life.

5. Moody, Dr. Raymond, *Life After Life,* New York: Bantam, 1975.

6. Paul, Russill, *The Yoga of Sound,* Novato, California, New World Library, 2004.

7. "Saccidananda Ashram." In Wikipedia. http://en.wikipedia.org/wiki/Saccidananda_Ashram.

8. Singh, Ravi and Brett, Ana. *Kundalini Yoga* DVD, White Lion Press, 2005.

9. Yogananda, Paramahansa, *Autobiography of a Yogi,* United States: The Philosophical Library, 1946.

YouTube Playlist

1. The Cosmic AUM (Harrison Graves)
https://www.youtube.com/watch?v=_7dSq8bJDgM&feature=youtu.be

2. The Chakra Mantras (Harrison Graves)
https://www.youtube.com/watch?v=zo7Si_eWbpA

3. The Ganesha Mantra (Harrison Graves)
https://www.youtube.com/watch?v=FyN7ewAh2l0

4. Triambakam Mantra (Harrison Graves)
https://www.youtube.com/watch?v=97efhU-U1Jc

5. OM Mani Padme Hum (Deva Premal)
https://www.youtube.com/watch?v=AUXfY5GOzgQ

6. The Long Time Sun (Snatam Kaur)
https://www.youtube.com/watch?v=T1D3ejwQiVg

7. Hey Ma Durga (Donna De Lory)
https://www.youtube.com/watch?v=Iwgu7dtaOHY

8. The Gayatri Mantra (Deva Premal)
https://www.youtube.com/watch?v=SlUsoWmso9U&list=RD7VsiKA6IS-I

9. Lokah Samastha (Deva Premal)
https://www.youtube.com/watch?v=usJl7oiZPnc

Made in the USA
Middletown, DE
12 May 2015